JUICING FOR BEGINNERS

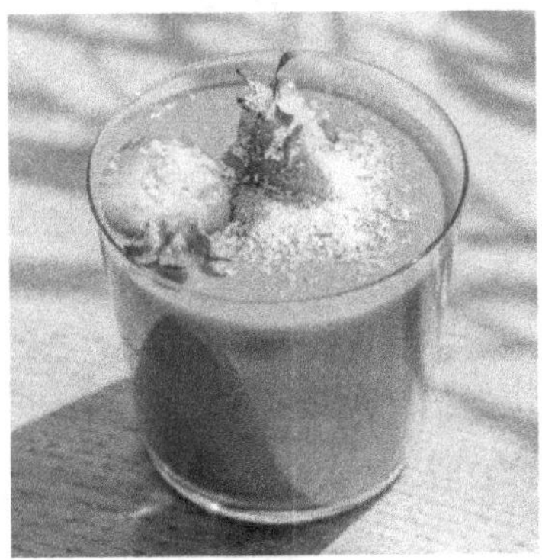

Your Path to a Refreshed Body and Mind with Healthy Drinks

Melissa Douglas

Table of contents

Introduction

Once upon a time, in a world bustling with the demands of modern life, there existed a humble yet powerful elixir that promised a path to vitality and well-being: the art of juicing. Our story begins not in a far-off land but right in the heart of everyday kitchens, where individuals sought a way to embrace health in a glass.

In the age of fast food and hectic schedules, the notion of juicing emerged as a beacon of hope for those yearning to reconnect with nature's bounty. The enchanting aroma of fresh fruits and vegetables wafted through the air, awakening a curiosity within the hearts of beginners eager to embark on this wholesome journey.

As the sun cast its warm glow on a kitchen counter adorned with an array of colorful produce, our protagonists, the budding juicers, stood at the threshold of a new adventure. The allure of radiant skin, increased energy, and a revitalized spirit beckoned them into the world of liquid nourishment.

The journey unfolded with the discovery of the benefits of juicing, a tale whispered by wellness enthusiasts and health gurus alike. From a boost in immune function to the promise of clearer skin, the protagonists were captivated by the magic contained within the vibrant juices they were about to create.

Guided by the desire for a healthier lifestyle, the beginners delved into the labyrinth of juicer options, navigating through the vast forest of centrifugal and masticating machines. Each juicer whispered its unique advantages, and the beginners, with wide-eyed wonder, began to understand that the choice of their juicing companion held the key to unlocking the full potential of their liquid journey.

As our intrepid beginners traversed the lush landscape of fruits, vegetables, and greens, they uncovered the secrets of crafting a symphony of flavors. From the sweet melody of ripe berries to the earthy undertones of leafy greens, they learned that juicing was not just a task but an art — a creative expression that could transform a mundane routine into a delightful ritual.

With the guidance of seasoned juicing alchemists, the beginners mastered the techniques of extracting liquid gold from nature's bounty. From the whirring sound of the juicer to the kaleidoscope of colors pouring into their glasses, the kitchen became a sanctuary of health and rejuvenation.

And so, the tale of juicing for beginners began, weaving a narrative of exploration, experimentation, and the discovery of the remarkable synergy between taste and well-being. As the beginners sipped on their first creations, a sense of empowerment blossomed within them, and they realized that this journey was not just about the juice but the transformation it brought to their lives.

And thus, dear reader, with the turning of each page, the story of juicing for beginners unfolds, inviting you to join the ranks of those who embraced this enchanting elixir and embarked on a quest for a healthier, more vibrant existence.

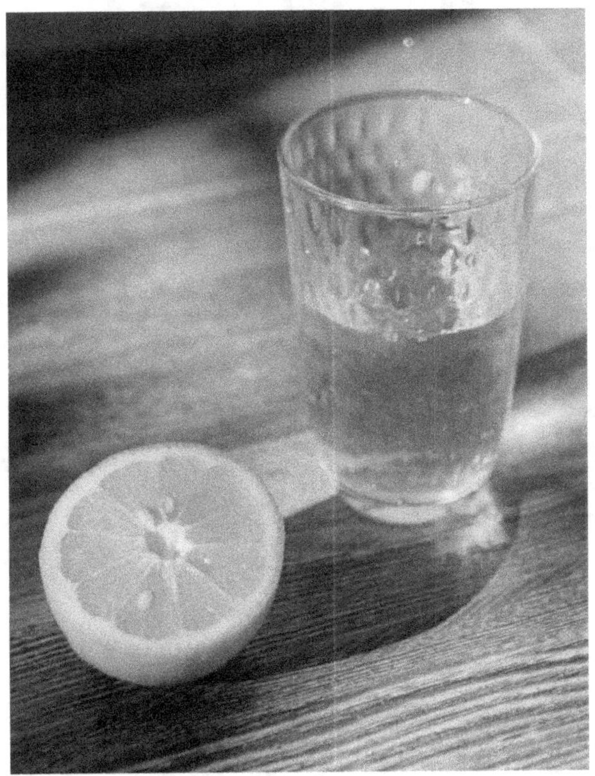

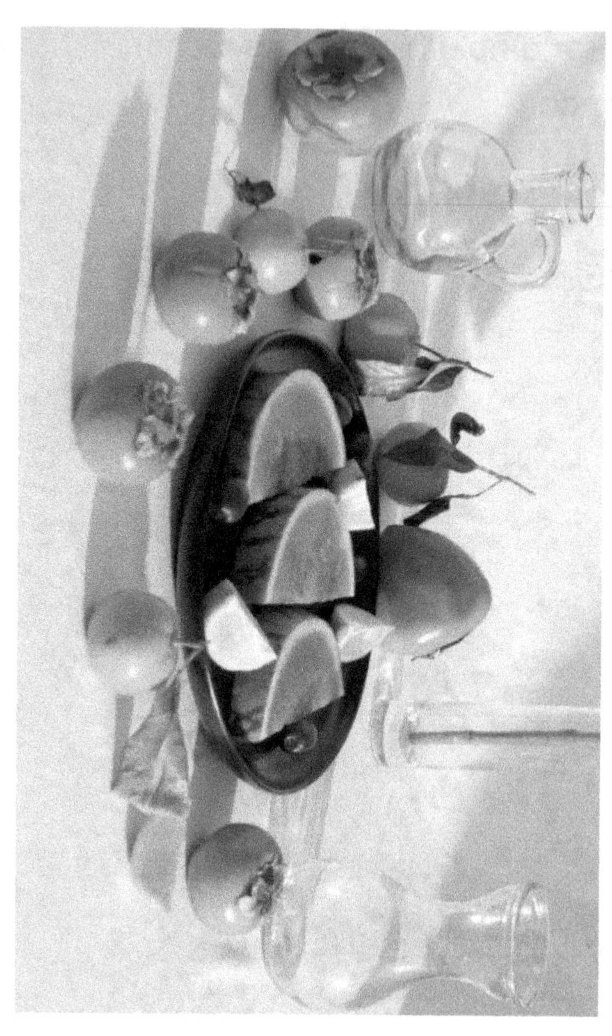

Chapter One

Juicing

Juicing is the process of extracting liquids from fruits and vegetables, typically using a juicer machine. This extraction separates the juice from the fibrous pulp, resulting in a concentrated liquid that contains vitamins, minerals, antioxidants, and other nutrients found in the product. The goal of juicing is to create a beverage that provides a quick and easily digestible source of essential nutrients, offering a convenient way to increase fruit and vegetable intake. Juicing can be enjoyed with a variety of fruits, vegetables, and greens, allowing for diverse flavor combinations and nutritional benefits.

Benefits Of Juicing

Juicing offers a myriad of benefits for

those seeking a refreshing approach to

a healthier lifestyle. Here are some key
advantages:

1. Increased Nutrient Absorption:
   Juicing extracts essential vitamins,
   minerals, and antioxidants from
   fruits and vegetables, providing a
   concentrated and easily
   absorbable form of nutrition.
2. Enhanced Hydration: Juices are
   an excellent source of hydration,
   especially when crafted from
   water-rich fruits and vegetables.
   Staying hydrated is crucial for
   overall health and well-being.
3. Supports Detoxification: Certain
   fruits and vegetables possess
   detoxifying properties, aiding the
   body in eliminating toxins. Juicing
   can contribute to a gentle and
   natural detox process.
4. Boosts Energy Levels: The high
   concentration of nutrients in fresh

juices can provide a natural energy boost, promoting alertness and vitality without the need for stimulants.

5. Improves Digestion: Juicing removes the insoluble fiber, making nutrients more easily digestible. This can be beneficial for individuals with sensitive digestive systems or those looking for a break from heavy fiber intake.

6. Promotes Weight Management: Including nutrient-dense juices in your diet can support weight management by providing essential nutrients while keeping calorie intake in check.

7. Clearer Skin: The abundance of vitamins and antioxidants in fruits and vegetables can contribute to healthier skin, promoting a radiant complexion and combating signs of aging.

8. Enhances Immune Function: Juices rich in vitamin C and other immune-boosting compounds can strengthen the immune system, helping the body ward off illnesses.

9. Encourages Variety in Diet: Juicing allows for the incorporation of a wide range of fruits and vegetables, promoting diversity in nutrients and flavors that may be challenging to achieve through whole foods alone.

10. Convenient Way to Consume Greens: For those who struggle to consume enough leafy greens, juicing provides an efficient and palatable method to include these nutrient-packed vegetables in their diet.

While juicing offers these benefits, it's essential to balance it with a well-rounded diet that includes whole fruits, vegetables, and other food groups for overall nutritional completeness.

Getting started with juicing

Embarking on the journey of juicing can be an exciting and healthful endeavor. Here's a guide to help you get started:

1. **Selecting a Juicer:**
   - Consider Types: Choose between centrifugal juicers (faster, more affordable) and masticating juicers (slower, better nutrient retention).

- Features: Look for easy cleaning, efficiency, and the ability to handle a variety of produce.

2. **Gathering Equipment:**
    - Juicer: Invest in a quality juicer based on your preferences and needs.
    - Cutting Board and Knife: For preparing fruits and vegetables.
    - Glass or Pitcher: To collect the juice.
    - Storage Containers: For any leftover juice.

3. **Choosing Ingredients:**

- Start Simple: Begin with familiar fruits and vegetables like apples, carrots, and cucumbers.

- Experiment: Gradually incorporate a variety of produce to explore different flavors and nutritional benefits.

- Fresh and Organic: Use fresh, preferably organic, produce for optimal taste and nutrient content.

4. **Basic Juicing Steps:**

- Wash Produce: Clean fruits and vegetables thoroughly.

- Prepare Ingredients: Peel (if necessary) and cut into manageable sizes.

- Juicing Process: Feed the produce through the juicer, collecting the extracted juice and separating it from the pulp.

- Stir and Serve: Give the juice a stir to mix any separated layers and enjoy immediately.

5. **Creating Balanced Recipes:**

- Mix Fruits and Vegetables: Combine sweet fruits with leafy greens for balanced flavors.

- Experiment with Ratios: Adjust the ratio of fruits to vegetables based on your taste preferences.

6. **Nutritional Tips:**

- Maximize Nutrient Intake: Include a variety of colored fruits and vegetables to ensure a broad spectrum of nutrients.

- Mind Sugar Content: Be mindful of high-sugar fruits; balance them with lower-sugar options.

7. **Juicing Plans:**

   - One-Week Beginner's Plan: Start with a simple plan to gradually incorporate juicing into your routine.

   - Customize: Tailor juicing plans based on your specific health goals and preferences.

8. **Cleaning and Maintenance:**

- Immediate Clean-up: Clean the juicer components immediately after use to prevent residues.

- Regular Maintenance: Follow the manufacturer's guidelines for routine maintenance to ensure your juicer's longevity.

9. **Delicious Juicing Recipes:**

- Energizing Citrus Blend: Oranges, grapefruits, and a hint of mint.

- Green Goddess Detox: Spinach, kale, cucumber, apple, and lemon.

10. **Staying Motivated:**

- Set Realistic Goals: Establish achievable juicing goals that align with your overall wellness objectives.

- Incorporate into Daily Routine: Make juicing a seamless part of your daily life.

11. **Troubleshooting:**

- Common Juicing Issues: Address common challenges like clogging, foaming, or uneven extraction.

- Solutions and Tips: Refer to troubleshooting sections in your juicer manual or seek advice from experienced juicers.

Remember, juicing is a personal and creative journey. Experiment with flavors, listen to your body, and enjoy the vibrant, healthful benefits of incorporating fresh, homemade juices into your lifestyle.

Chapter Two

Criteria to consider when selecting the right juicer

Selecting the right juicer involves considering various criteria to ensure it meets your preferences, needs, and lifestyle. Here are key factors to consider:

1. **Type of Juicer:**
   - Centrifugal Juicers:
     - *Pros:* Quick juicing, generally more affordable.

- - *Cons:* May generate heat, potentially affecting nutrient content.
- Masticating Juicers (Cold-Press):
  - *Pros:* Operate at slower speeds, preserving more nutrients and enzymes.
  - *Cons:* Generally more expensive, slower juicing process.

2. **Ease of Use and Cleaning:**

- User-Friendly Design: Opt for a juicer with a straightforward assembly and operation.

- Easy to Clean: Look for
  components that are easy to
  disassemble and clean, as this
  encourages regular use.

3. **Durability and Build Quality:**

- Material: Choose a juicer with
  durable, high-quality materials that
  can withstand regular use.
- Motor Power: Consider a juicer
  with a robust motor to handle a
  variety of produce.

4. **Juicing Speed:**

- Variable Speed Settings: Some juicers offer adjustable speeds for different types of produce. This can be beneficial for optimizing extraction.

5. **Noise Level:**

- Quiet Operation: If noise is a concern, look for juicers designed for quieter performance.

6. **Juice Yield:**

- Efficiency: Consider the juicer's ability to extract maximum juice from fruits and vegetables, minimizing waste.

7. **Pulp Adjustment:**

- Pulp Control Feature: Some juicers allow you to adjust the level of pulp in your juice, providing flexibility based on personal preference.

8. **Size and Storage:**

- Compact Design: Especially important if you have limited kitchen space.
- Vertical or Horizontal Orientation: Vertical juicers are often more space-efficient.

9. **Price and Budget:**

- Affordability: Determine your budget and look for juicers that offer the best value within that range.

10. **Brand Reputation and Reviews:**

- Research Brands: Look for reputable brands with positive customer reviews to ensure reliability and customer satisfaction.

11. **Versatility:**

- Multifunctionality: Some juicers can handle a variety of tasks, such as making nut butter or sorbets.

Consider if additional functions
align with your needs.

12. **Warranty:**

- Coverage: Check the warranty period to ensure protection against defects and potential issues.

13. **Cleaning and Maintenance:**

- Dishwasher-Friendly Parts: Dishwasher-safe components can simplify the cleaning process.
- Ease of Maintenance: Consider the overall maintenance requirements outlined by the manufacturer.

14. **Customer Support:**

- Availability: Ensure that the manufacturer provides adequate customer support and resources for troubleshooting.

By carefully considering these criteria, you can select a juicer that aligns with your lifestyle, preferences, and juicing goals, enhancing your overall experience and satisfaction with the appliance.

Types of Juicers

There are several types of juicers available in the market, each with its own method of extracting juice from fruits and vegetables. Here are the main types:

1. **Centrifugal Juicers:**
   - How They Work: These juicers use a high-speed spinning blade to chop and break down produce, separating the juice from the pulp through centrifugal force.
   - Pros:
     - Fast juicing process.
     - Generally more affordable.
   - Cons:

- May generate heat, potentially affecting nutrient content.
    - Might produce less juice compared to other types.

2. Masticating Juicers (Cold-Press or Slow Juicers):

- How They Work: Masticating juicers use a slower, crushing and squeezing action to extract juice. This method is thought to preserve more nutrients and enzymes.
- Pros:
    - Higher juice yield.

- Preserves more nutrients due to the slower extraction process.
    - Suitable for juicing leafy greens and soft fruits.
- Cons:
    - Slower juicing process.
    - Generally more expensive.

3. **Twin-Gear (Triturating) Juicers:**

- How They Work: These juicers have two interlocking gears that crush and grind produce, effectively extracting juice.

- Pros:

  - High juice yield.

  - Efficient at juicing various types of produce, including leafy greens.

- Cons:

  - Typically more expensive.

  - Cleaning can be more intricate.

4. **Vertical Juicers:**

- How They Work: Vertical juicers have a space-saving design where the auger is oriented vertically.

- Pros:

- - Compact and requires less counter space.
  - Often easy to assemble and clean.
- Cons:
  - May have a slightly smaller chute, requiring more preparation of produce.

5. **Citrus Juicers:**

- How They Work: Specifically designed for citrus fruits, these juicers typically have a cone-shaped reamer to extract juice.
- Pros:

- ○ Efficient for juicing citrus fruits like oranges, lemons, and limes.
  - ○ Simple to use.
- Cons:
  - ○ Limited to citrus fruits only.

6. **Manual Juicers:**

- How They Work: Operated by hand, manual juicers can be simple reamers, hand-cranked devices, or lever-style juicers.
- Pros:
  - ○ No reliance on electricity.
  - ○ Can be portable.
- Cons:

- o Requires physical effort.
- o Generally not as efficient as electric juicers.

7. **Hydraulic Press Juicers:**

- How They Work: These juicers use hydraulic pressure to extract juice from produce, often in combination with a two-step process involving grinding and pressing.
- Pros:
  - o High juice yield.
  - o Preserves nutrients well.
- Cons:

- o Typically larger and more expensive.
- o Cleaning may be more involved.

When choosing a juicer, consider your juicing preferences, the types of produce you plan to juice, ease of cleaning, and your budget. Each type has its own set of advantages and limitations, so selecting the right juicer depends on your specific needs and priorities.

Chapter Three

Essential ingredients for juicing

Essential Ingredients for Juicing: Fruits, Vegetables, Herbs, and Greens

Juicing is a vibrant celebration of nature's bounty, offering a rainbow of flavors and an abundance of nutrients. Here's a comprehensive guide to essential ingredients, categorized into fruits, vegetables, herbs, and greens, to elevate your juicing experience:

1. **Fruits:**

A. Citrus Fruits:

- Oranges: Bursting with vitamin C and a sweet, tangy flavor.

- Grapefruits: Refreshing and known for their citrusy zing.

- Lemons/Limes: Add a bright, citrusy kick to your juices.

B. Berries:

- Strawberries: Sweet and packed with antioxidants.

- Blueberries: Rich in anthocyanins for a deep color and health benefits.

- Raspberries/Blackberries: Provide a delightful tartness.

C. Tropical Fruits:

- Pineapple: Sweet and aids digestion with its enzyme bromelain.

- Mango: Creamy texture and a tropical sweetness.

- Kiwi: Adds a unique flavor and is high in vitamin C.

D. Stone Fruits:

- Peaches: Juicy and sweet with a fragrant aroma.

- Plums: Offer a balance of sweetness and tartness.

- Apricots: Provide a delicate sweetness.

2. **Vegetables:**

A. Root Vegetables:

- Carrots: Sweet and vibrant orange color, high in beta-carotene.

- Beets: Earthy with a beautiful deep red hue.

- Sweet Potatoes: Nutrient-rich and add sweetness to juices.

B. Leafy Greens:

- Spinach: Mild flavor, rich in iron and vitamins.

- Kale: Robust and nutrient-dense, a powerhouse of vitamins.

- Swiss Chard: Colorful stems and leaves, high in antioxidants.

C. Cucumbers and Celery:

- Cucumbers: Hydrating and add a refreshing element.

- Celery: Crisp and mild, contributes to overall hydration.

D. Bell Peppers:

- Red, Yellow, Green: Add sweetness and vibrant colors.

3. **Herbs:**

A. Mint:

- Spearmint/Peppermint: Refreshing and can enhance the overall flavor.

B. Basil:

- Sweet Basil: Adds a hint of sweetness and complements fruits well.

C. Cilantro/Coriander:

- Cilantro: Fresh and citrusy, pairs well with various ingredients.

4. **Greens:**

A. Wheatgrass:

- Nutrient-Rich: Packed with vitamins, minerals, and antioxidants.

B. Kale and Spinach:

- Kale: A nutritional powerhouse with a slightly earthy taste.
- Spinach: Mild flavor and high in iron and folate.

C. Swiss Chard and Collard Greens:

- Swiss Chard: Colorful stems and a mild, slightly sweet taste.
- Collard Greens: Robust and rich in nutrients.

Tips for Juicing Ingredients:

1. Balance: Mix sweet fruits with leafy greens for a balanced flavor profile.

2. Experiment: Try different combinations to discover your favorite blends.

3. Preparation: Wash and prep ingredients before juicing for efficiency.

4. Incorporate Variety: Rotate ingredients to ensure a broad spectrum of nutrients.

Juicing offers a canvas for creativity and nourishment. Combine these essential ingredients to craft delicious, nutrient-packed juices that invigorate your body and delight your taste buds.

5. Hydration Boost: Include water-rich fruits like watermelon or cucumber to enhance the hydrating qualities of your juices.

6. Texture and Thickness: Adjust the texture by adding ingredients like bananas for thickness or watery fruits like apples for a lighter consistency.

7. Color Palette: Embrace a diverse color palette to signify a variety of nutrients. Vibrant colors often indicate a range of antioxidants and phytochemicals.

8. Seasonal Selections: Incorporate seasonal produce for freshness

and optimal flavor. Seasonal ingredients are often more cost-effective and locally sourced.

9. Freeze Fruits: Freeze fruits like berries or grapes beforehand to add a chilled and refreshing element to your juices, especially during warmer months.

10. Juicing Greens: Roll leafy greens into compact bundles before juicing to optimize extraction efficiency.

11. Citrus Zest: Add a burst of flavor by incorporating the zest of citrus fruits. The peel contains essential oils that can enhance taste.

12.   Ginger and Turmeric: Infuse

your juices with these potent

anti-inflammatory roots for added

health benefits and a zesty kick.

13.   Customization: Tailor your

juices to suit your taste

preferences and dietary goals.

Adjust sweetness or acidity levels

based on personal preference.

14.   Juice Storage: Consume

freshly juiced beverages

immediately for maximum

nutrition. If storing, use airtight

containers and refrigerate for up to

24-48 hours.

Delicious Juicing Recipes:

1. **Energizing Citrus Blend:**
   - Oranges, Grapefruits, Lemons
   - Carrots
   - Ginger (small piece)

2. **Green Goddess Detox:**
   - Kale
   - Cucumbers
   - Green Apples
   - Celery
   - Lemon

3. **Tropical Paradise Smoothie:**
   - Pineapple
   - Mango

- Coconut Water

- Spinach

4. **Berry Bliss Explosion:**
   - Blueberries

   - Raspberries

   - Strawberries

   - Greek Yogurt (optional for creaminess)

Juicing techniques

Mastering juicing techniques is crucial to extract the maximum goodness from your chosen ingredients. Here's a guide to help you navigate the juicing process effectively:

1. **Prepare Your Ingredients:**

   - Wash all fruits, vegetables, herbs, and greens thoroughly to remove dirt and pesticides.
   - Peel fruits and vegetables if desired, especially if they have thick or bitter skins.

2. **Cut Ingredients Into Manageable Pieces:**

   - Slice larger fruits and vegetables into smaller chunks that fit easily into the juicer chute.
   - For leafy greens, roll them into compact bundles to optimize extraction.

3. **Operate Your Juicer:**

   - Follow the specific instructions in your juicer's manual for assembly and operation.
   - Ensure the machine is properly set up, and safety mechanisms are engaged.

4. **Sequential Juicing:**

- If using a variety of ingredients, alternate between harder and softer items to facilitate efficient juicing.

5. **Leafy Greens Technique:**

- For greens like spinach or kale, tightly roll them into a compact bundle before feeding into the juicer. This helps maximize juice extraction.

6. **Use the Plunger:**

- Utilize the plunger (if provided) to gently guide ingredients into the juicer chute, ensuring a steady and controlled feed.

7. **Pulp Management:**

- Monitor the pulp collection
  container and empty it as needed
  to prevent clogging.
- Some juicers have adjustable
  settings for pulp extraction,
  allowing you to customize the pulp
  level in your juice.

8. **Juice Separation:**

- After juicing, give the juice a
  gentle stir to mix any separated
  layers and ensure an even flavor.

9. **Immediate Consumption:**

- Freshly juiced beverages are at
  their nutritional peak. Consume
  them immediately for maximum
  benefits.

10. **Clean Your Juicer Promptly:**

- Disassemble the juicer and clean each part as soon as possible after use to prevent residues from drying and becoming challenging to remove.
- Follow the manufacturer's cleaning instructions.

11. **Experiment with Combinations:**

- Be creative and try different ingredient combinations to discover flavors that suit your taste preferences.

12. **Adjust for Texture:**

- If you prefer a thicker juice, include ingredients like bananas or avocados. For a lighter consistency, incorporate watery fruits like apples or cucumbers.

13. **Incorporate Citrus Wisely:**

- Citrus fruits can add zest to your juice, but a little goes a long way. Start with small amounts and adjust to taste.

14. Prevent Foam:

- If foam is undesirable, try skimming it off the top of your juice or let it settle before consuming.

15. Cleanup Tips:

- Rinse components immediately after use to prevent stubborn stains.
- Periodically deep clean your juicer by following the manufacturer's guidelines.

16. Repurpose Pulp:

- Get creative with leftover pulp by using it in recipes like muffins, soups, or composting for minimal waste.

17. **Explore Temperature Variations:**

- Experiment with chilled ingredients or ice cubes for a refreshing, cold-pressed experience.

By honing these juicing techniques, you'll not only maximize the nutritional benefits of your juices but also enhance your overall juicing experience. Whether you're a beginner or an experienced juicer, these tips can elevate your skills and allow you to savor the full spectrum of flavors in every glass.

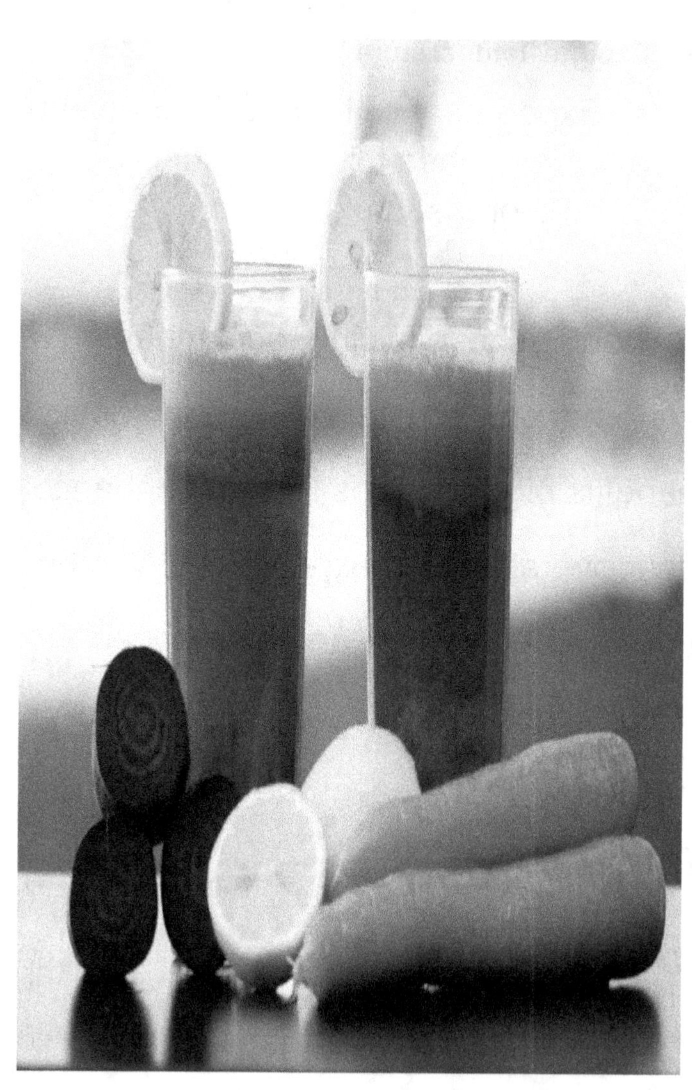

Chapter Four

Basic juicing steps

Juicing can be a straightforward and enjoyable process when you follow these basic steps:

1. **Gather Your Ingredients:**

   - Select a variety of fresh fruits, vegetables, herbs, and greens based on your taste preferences and nutritional goals.

2. **Wash and Prepare:**

   - Wash all produce thoroughly to remove dirt and pesticides.
   - Peel fruits and vegetables if desired, especially if they have thick or bitter skins.
   - Cut larger items into manageable pieces.

3. **Set Up Your Juicer:**

- Refer to your juicer's manual for specific assembly instructions.
- Ensure the machine is placed on a stable surface, and safety mechanisms are engaged.

4. **Turn On the Juicer:**

- Power up your juicer and make sure it's running smoothly before adding ingredients.

5. **Sequential Juicing:**

- Alternate between harder and softer ingredients to optimize the juicing process.
- For example, follow a leafy green with a cucumber or apple.

6. **Feed Ingredients Into the Chute:**

- Use the plunger (if provided) to gently guide ingredients into the juicer chute.

- Avoid overloading the chute to prevent clogging.

7. **Collect the Juice:**

   - Position a glass or pitcher under the juice spout to collect the extracted liquid.
   - Monitor the juice container to prevent overflow.

8. **Observe Pulp Collection:**

   - Keep an eye on the pulp container and empty it as needed to avoid clogging.
   - Adjust the juicer settings for preferred pulp levels if available.

9. **Stir the Juice:**

   - After juicing is complete, give the juice a gentle stir to mix any separated layers and ensure an even flavor.

10. **Immediate Consumption:**

- Freshly juiced beverages are at their nutritional peak. Consume them immediately to maximize benefits.

11. **Cleaning:**

- Disassemble the juicer and clean each part as soon as possible after use.
- Rinse components under running water and use a brush (if provided) to remove any residues.
- Follow the manufacturer's cleaning instructions.

12. **Store or Enjoy:**

- If you're not consuming the juice immediately, store it in an airtight container in the refrigerator.
- Some juices can separate over time, so give it a quick stir before drinking.

13. **Experiment and Customize:**

- Experiment with different ingredient combinations to discover flavors that suit your taste preferences.
- Adjust the ratio of fruits to vegetables based on your desired sweetness level.

14. **Stay Hydrated:**

- Juicing can contribute to your daily hydration. Consider it as a refreshing addition to your fluid intake.

By following these basic juicing steps, you'll be well on your way to creating delicious and nutritious beverages that align with your health and wellness goals. As you become more comfortable with the process, feel free to experiment and tailor your recipes to your unique taste preferences.

Creating balance recipes

Creating balanced juicing recipes involves combining a variety of fruits, vegetables, herbs, and greens to ensure a harmonious blend of flavors, textures, and nutrients. Here's a guide to help you achieve balance in your juice creations:

1. **Include a Variety of Colors:**
   - Different colors often indicate varying nutrients. Incorporate a mix of vibrant hues for a broad spectrum of health benefits.

2. **Sweet and Tart Balance:**

- Balance sweet fruits like apples, oranges, or mangoes with tart options such as berries, lemons, or pomegranates.

3. **Leafy Greens and Vegetables:**

- Integrate nutrient-dense leafy greens like kale, spinach, or Swiss chard.
- Add vegetables like cucumber, celery, or carrots for additional vitamins and minerals.

4. **Herbs for Flavor Enhancement:**

- Include herbs like mint, basil, or cilantro to elevate the overall flavor profile without adding excessive calories.

5. **Citrus Zest for Zing:**

- Add zest from citrus fruits to provide a refreshing and zesty kick to your juice.

6. Experiment with Root Vegetables:

- Incorporate root vegetables like beets or sweet potatoes for earthy flavors and added nutritional benefits.

7. Texture Variety:

- Combine fruits that offer different textures, such as the creaminess of bananas or avocados with the juiciness of watermelon or pineapple.

8. Consider Aromatics:

- Explore aromatic ingredients like ginger or turmeric for a unique and fragrant element in your juice.

9. **Balanced Sugar Content:**

- Be mindful of the sugar content in your juice. Balance sweet fruits with lower-sugar options to create a beverage that aligns with your dietary preferences.

10. **Hydrating Components:**

- Include hydrating ingredients like cucumber or watermelon for a refreshing and thirst-quenching quality.

11. **Experiment with Nut Milks:**

- Consider adding a splash of nut milk (such as almond or coconut) for creaminess and an extra layer of flavor.

12. **Ratio Adjustments:**

- Adjust the ratio of fruits to vegetables based on your taste preferences. Gradually increase the vegetable content as you become accustomed to the flavors.

13. **Mindful Sweeteners:**

- If additional sweetness is desired, consider natural sweeteners like honey or agave syrup in moderation.

14. **Create Theme-Based Recipes:**

- Explore themes such as tropical, citrusy, or green detox to guide your ingredient choices.

15. **Keep It Simple:**

- Sometimes, simplicity is key. A few well-chosen ingredients can create a balanced and delicious juice.

16. **Nutrient-Rich Additions:**

- Boost nutritional content by adding ingredients like chia seeds, flaxseeds, or spirulina.

17. **Listen to Your Taste Buds:**

- Your taste preferences matter. Experiment, taste as you go, and adjust ingredients to suit your palate.

18. **Record Your Recipes:**

- Note down successful combinations for future reference and to track your favorite recipes.

Creating balanced juice recipes is both an art and a science. As you experiment and fine-tune your creations, you'll discover delightful blends that not only tantalize your taste buds but also contribute to your overall well-being.

Nutritional tips: the maximizing nutrient intake and understanding sugar contents

Nutritional Tips for Juicing:

1. **Maximize Nutrient Intake:**
   - Diverse Ingredients: Include a variety of fruits, vegetables, herbs, and greens to ensure a broad spectrum of nutrients.
   - Colorful Palette: Opt for vibrant colors, as different pigments often

signify various beneficial
compounds.

- Leafy Greens: Incorporate
  nutrient-dense leafy greens like
  kale, spinach, or Swiss chard for
  vitamins and minerals.

2. **Mindful Pairing:**

- Balance Sweet and Savory:
  Combine sweet fruits with less
  sugary vegetables to strike a
  balance in taste and nutritional
  content.
- Citrus Addition: Citrus fruits can
  enhance flavor while contributing
  vitamin C and antioxidants.

3. **Include Nutrient-Rich Additions:**

- Seeds and Nuts: Add chia seeds, flaxseeds, or nuts for an extra boost of omega-3 fatty acids, protein, and fiber.

- Superfoods: Experiment with nutrient-rich additions like spirulina, wheatgrass, or turmeric.

4. **Hydration Boost:**

- Watery Fruits and Vegetables: Include hydrating ingredients like cucumber, watermelon, or celery for an extra dose of hydration.

- Coconut Water: Use coconut water as a base for added electrolytes.

5. **Watch the Sugar Content:**

- Mindful Fruit Selection: Be aware of the natural sugars in fruits. Choose lower-sugar options like berries, kiwi, or green apples.

- Limit High-Sugar Fruits: Moderation is key when incorporating high-sugar fruits like mangoes or pineapples to manage sugar intake.

6. **Add Healthy Fats:**

- Avocado: Include avocado for creaminess and healthy fats.

- Nut Milks: Use almond or coconut milk for a dose of healthy fats and added flavor.

7. **Control Portion Sizes:**

- Balanced Ratios: Aim for a balanced ratio of fruits to vegetables. Gradually increase vegetable content as your palate adjusts.

- Caloric Awareness: Be mindful of caloric content, especially if you are incorporating many high-calorie ingredients.

8. **Include Fiber-Rich Pulp:**

- Reuse Pulp: Repurpose leftover pulp in recipes like soups, stews, or baked goods to retain fiber content and minimize waste.

9. **Rotate Ingredients:**

- Seasonal Variety: Incorporate seasonal produce for freshness and potentially increased nutrient content.

- Avoid Monotony: Rotate ingredients to prevent nutrient deficiencies and keep your taste buds engaged.

10. **Consider Nutritional Goals:**

- Fitness Goals: Adjust your juice recipes based on specific fitness or health goals, whether it's weight loss, muscle building, or overall well-being.

11. **Consult a Nutritionist:**

- Personalized Advice: If you have specific dietary concerns or health conditions, consult with a nutritionist for personalized guidance on juicing.

12. **Post-Juice Meal Planning:**

- Balanced Diet: Ensure your overall diet is balanced by incorporating a mix of proteins, carbohydrates, healthy fats, and other nutrients outside of juicing.

13. **Juicing Plans:**

- One-Week Plans: Consider short-term juicing plans to kickstart

a healthier lifestyle, but always
incorporate whole foods for
long-term sustainability.

14. **Educate Yourself:**

- Nutritional Knowledge: Stay
  informed about the nutritional
  content of different ingredients to
  make informed choices when
  creating your juices.

Remember, juicing should complement
a well-rounded and diverse diet. While
juicing offers a convenient way to boost
nutrient intake, it's essential to maintain
overall dietary balance for optimal
health.

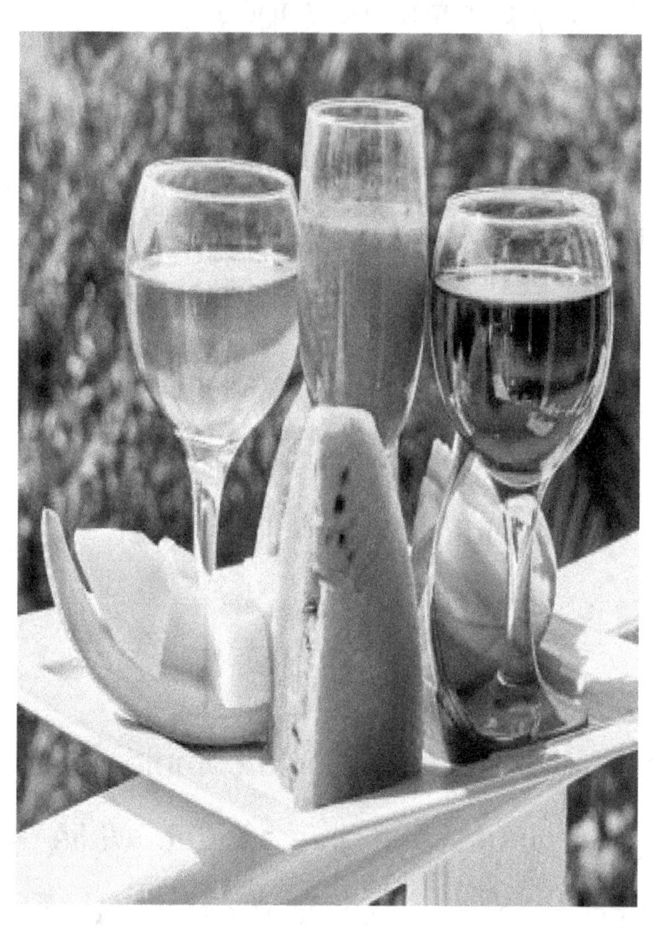

Chapter Five

Juicing plan

One-week beginner's plan

One-Week Beginner's Juicing Plan:

Day 1: Citrus Burst

- Morning:
    - 2 Oranges
    - 1 Grapefruit
- Midday:
    - 2 Carrots
    - 1 Apple
- Afternoon:
    - Handful of Spinach
    - 1 Cucumber
- Evening:

- 1 Lemon (with peel, if organic)

Day 2: Green Vitality

- Morning:
    - 2 Green Apples
    - Handful of Kale
- Midday:
    - 1 Cucumber
    - 1 Celery stalk
- Afternoon:
    - 1 Kiwi
    - Handful of Spinach
- Evening:
    - Small piece of Ginger

Day 3: Berry Bliss

- Morning:

    - Handful of Blueberries

    - 1 Banana

- Midday:

    - 1 Cup Strawberries

    - 1 Apple

- Afternoon:

    - Handful of Raspberries

    - 1 Carrot

- Evening:

    - 1 Lime

Day 4: Refreshing Hydration

- Morning:

    - 1 Cucumber

    - 1 Apple

- Midday:

- o 1 Orange
- o 1 Carrot
- **Afternoon:**
  - o Handful of Mint Leaves
  - o 1 Lemon
- **Evening:**
  - o 1/2 Watermelon (remove seeds)

Day 5: Tropical Paradise

- **Morning:**
  - o 1 Mango
  - o 1 Banana
- **Midday:**
  - o 1 Cup Pineapple chunks
  - o Handful of Spinach
- **Afternoon:**

- - 1 Kiwi
  - 1 Carrot
- Evening:
  - 1/2 Coconut (water and flesh)

Day 6: Rooted Energy
- Morning:
  - 2 Beets (peeled)
  - 1 Apple
- Midday:
  - 1 Carrot
  - Handful of Spinach
- Afternoon:
  - 1 Orange
  - Small piece of Ginger
- Evening:

- 1 Lemon

Day 7: Citrus-Pineapple Delight

- Morning:

    - 1 Orange

    - 1 Cup Pineapple chunks

- Midday:

    - 1 Banana

    - 1 Carrot

- Afternoon:

    - 1 Grapefruit

    - Handful of Spinach

- Evening:

    - 1 Lime

Tips for the Week:

- Hydration: To keep hydrated, drink plenty of water throughout the day.

- Portion Control: Be mindful of serving sizes and attentive to your body's signals of hunger and fullness.

- Variety: Experiment with ingredient combinations to keep your taste buds engaged.

- Adjust to Taste: Feel free to adjust the quantity of ingredients based on your taste preferences.

- Whole Foods: Complement your juices with whole foods for a well-rounded diet.

This one-week beginner's juicing plan is designed to introduce a variety of flavors and nutrients to your routine. Remember to listen to your body, enjoy the process, and gradually incorporate juicing into your overall lifestyle.

Customizing for goals

Customizing Juicing Plan for Specific Goals:

Goal: Weight Loss

- Morning:
    - 1 Grapefruit (metabolism booster)

- - 2 Celery stalks (low-calorie
    hydrator)
- Midday:
  - 1 Cucumber (low-calorie
    base)
  - Handful of Spinach
    (nutrient-rich)
- Afternoon:
  - 1 Green Apple (fiber for
    satiety)
  - 1 Lemon (digestive aid)
- Evening:
  - 1/2 Beet (natural detoxifier)
  - Small piece of Ginger
    (metabolism booster)

Goal: Muscle Building

- Morning:
  - 1 Banana (energy boost)
  - 1/2 Avocado (healthy fats)
- Midday:
  - Handful of Blueberries (antioxidants)
  - 1 Carrot (beta-carotene for recovery)
- Afternoon:
  - 1 Cup Pineapple chunks (anti-inflammatory)
  - Handful of Kale (iron and calcium)
- Evening:
  - 1/2 Cup Greek Yogurt (protein)

- Small piece of Turmeric (anti-inflammatory)

- Morning:
  - 1 Lemon (alkalizing)
  - Handful of Mint Leaves (digestive aid)
- Midday:
  - 1 Cucumber (hydrating)
  - 1/2 Beet (liver support)
- Afternoon:
  - 1 Cup Kale (chlorophyll-rich)
  - 1 Lime (cleansing)
- Evening:
  - 1/2 Cup Aloe Vera Juice (detoxifying)

- ○ Small piece of Ginger (anti-inflammatory)

Goal: Immune Support

- Morning:
  - ○ 1 Orange (vitamin C)
  - ○ 1/2 Cup Berries (antioxidants)
- Midday:
  - ○ 1 Carrot (beta-carotene)
  - ○ 1/2 Beet (immune support)
- Afternoon:
  - ○ 1 Kiwi (vitamin K)
  - ○ Handful of Spinach (iron)
- Evening:
  - ○ 1/2 Lemon (vitamin C)

- Small piece of Turmeric (anti-inflammatory)

Goal: Energy Boost
- Morning:
  - 1 Apple (natural sugars for quick energy)
  - Handful of Spinach (iron for energy production)
- Midday:
  - 1 Banana (potassium for energy)
  - 1/2 Avocado (healthy fats)
- Afternoon:
  - 1/2 Cup Pineapple chunks (natural sugars)

- o 1 Cup Coconut Water
    (electrolytes)
- Evening:
  - o 1/2 Cup Greek Yogurt
    (protein for sustained
    energy)
  - o Small piece of Ginger
    (metabolism booster)

Tips for Customization:

- Adjust portion sizes based on your
  caloric needs.
- Experiment with ingredient
  combinations to suit your taste
  preferences.

- Include a mix of fruits, vegetables, herbs, and greens for diverse nutrients.
- Stay hydrated with water throughout the day.
- Consider consulting a nutritionist for personalized advice.

Customizing your juicing plan based on specific goals allows you to tailor your nutrient intake to support your unique health objectives. Listen to your body's responses and make adjustments as needed to achieve the desired outcomes.

Troubleshooting

Common Juicing Issues and Solutions:

1. Juicer Clogging:

- Issue: Fibrous or dense fruits and vegetables can lead to juicer clogs.

- Solution: Cut produce into smaller pieces, alternate between soft and hard ingredients, and clean the juicer regularly during juicing sessions.

2. Excessive Foam:

- Issue: Certain fruits and vegetables, especially citrus, can create excessive foam.

- Solution: Skim off the foam using a spoon or let the juice sit for a while to allow the foam to settle. You can also strain the juice to remove foam before consumption.

3. Juice Separation:

- Issue: Different densities of ingredients can cause the juice to separate.

- Solution: Stir the juice thoroughly before consuming. Consider choosing ingredients with similar textures to minimize separation.

4. Pulp Too Wet or Too Dry:

- Issue: Inconsistent pulp texture can indicate juicer inefficiency.

- Solution: Adjust the juicer settings if available. For wet pulp, increase extraction time; for dry pulp, reduce it. Ensure the juicer is clean and properly assembled.

5. Overheating:

- Issue: Continuous juicing can lead to overheating in some juicers.

- Solution: Allow the juicer to cool down between batches. If juicing large quantities, consider pausing to prevent overheating.

6. Difficulty Juicing Leafy Greens:

- Issue: Leafy greens may not be effectively juiced in certain machines.

- Solution: Bundle leafy greens tightly before feeding them into the juicer. Consider using a masticating or triturating juicer, which is more efficient with greens.

7. Too Bitter or Earthy Flavor:

- Issue: Certain greens or roots can contribute to a bitter or earthy taste.

- Solution: Balance bitter flavors with sweeter fruits. Experiment with citrus, apples, or carrots to

enhance sweetness and mask
bitterness.

8. High Sugar Content:

- Issue: Some fruits are high in
  natural sugars, leading to a
  calorie-dense juice.

- Solution: Be mindful of high-sugar
  fruits and balance them with
  low-sugar options. Consider
  diluting with water or incorporating
  more vegetables.

9. Cleaning Challenges:

- Issue: Juicers can be challenging
  to clean, deterring regular use.

- Solution: Clean your juicer immediately after use. Consider juicers with dishwasher-safe parts for convenience. Follow the manufacturer's cleaning instructions.

10. Oxidation:

- Issue: Exposure to air can lead to oxidation and nutrient loss.
- Solution: Consume juice immediately after preparation for maximum nutritional benefits. Store in airtight containers and refrigerate if necessary.

11. Lack of Variety:

- Issue: Sticking to the same ingredients can lead to taste fatigue and nutrient imbalance.

- Solution: Experiment with a variety of fruits, vegetables, herbs, and greens. Rotate ingredients to ensure a diverse nutrient profile.

12. Ignoring Seasonality:

- Issue: Not considering seasonal produce can affect freshness and cost.

- Solution: Choose fruits and vegetables that are in-season for optimal freshness, taste, and cost-effectiveness.

13. Not Drinking Enough Water:

- Issue: Relying solely on juices may lead to dehydration.

- Solution: Drink plenty of water alongside your juices to maintain proper hydration levels.

Addressing these common juicing issues and implementing the suggested solutions can enhance your juicing experience, making it more enjoyable and effective.

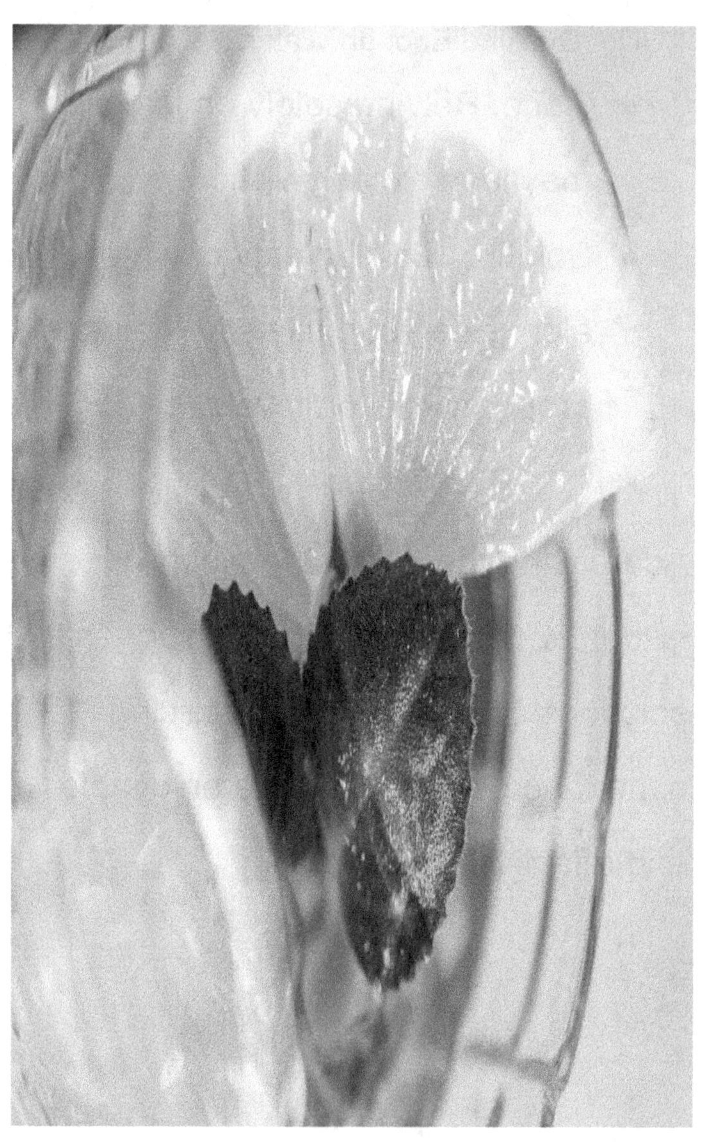

Chapter Six

Cleaning and maintenance of juicer

Proper Cleaning and Maintenance of Your Juicer:

Cleaning Steps:

1. Unplug the Juicer:
   - Always start by unplugging your juicer to ensure safety during the cleaning process.
2. Disassemble the Juicer:
   - Take apart the juicer components as per the manufacturer's instructions. Remove the pulp collector,

juice container, and any

removable parts.

3. Empty and Dispose of Pulp:

   ○ Dispose of the extracted

   pulp. You can use it in

   recipes, compost, or discard

   it based on your preference.

4. Rinse Components:

   ○ Rinse each removable

   component under running

   water immediately after use

   to prevent residues from

   drying and becoming harder

   to clean.

5. Use a Soft Brush:

   ○ If your juicer comes with a

   brush, use it to gently scrub

the mesh screen, cutting
blades, and other parts.
Take care not to harm any
sensitive parts.

6. Soak Removable Parts:

   o Soak removable parts, such
     as the mesh screen, in warm
     soapy water for a few
     minutes to loosen any
     remaining pulp or residue.

7. Clean Tricky Spots:

   o Pay attention to areas that
     may trap pulp, such as
     crevices and corners. A soft
     brush or toothbrush can be
     useful for cleaning these
     spots.

8. Deep Cleaning as Needed:

   ○ Periodically perform a deep
   clean by disassembling your
   juicer and cleaning each part
   thoroughly. Refer to your
   juicer's manual for guidance
   on deep cleaning
   procedures.

9. Check for Residue:

   ○ Inspect each part to ensure
   no residues or pulp are left
   behind. This is especially
   important for the mesh
   screen and cutting blades.

10. Dry Components:

   ○ After cleaning, thoroughly
   dry each component before

reassembling the juicer.
Air-dry or use a clean, dry
cloth to avoid any moisture
buildup.

Maintenance Tips:

1. Regular Inspection:

    ○ Periodically inspect your
    juicer for signs of wear and
    tear. Check the blades,
    mesh screen, and other
    parts for any damage.

2. Sharpen Blades:

    ○ If your juicer has cutting
    blades, check them for
    dullness. Follow the
    manufacturer's instructions

for safely sharpening or
replacing blades if needed.

3. Lubricate Moving Parts:

   o If your juicer has moving
     parts, lubricate them as per
     the manufacturer's
     recommendations to
     maintain smooth operation.

4. Avoid Overloading:

   o Follow the recommended
     capacity guidelines for your
     juicer to avoid overloading,
     which can lead to strain on
     the motor and reduced
     efficiency.

5. Clean Immediately:

- Clean your juicer immediately after each use to prevent residues from hardening and becoming difficult to remove.

6. Store Properly:

- When not in use, store your juice in a dry and cool place. To shield it from dust, try to keep it covered.

7. Follow Manufacturer Guidelines:

- Always follow the cleaning and maintenance guidelines provided by the manufacturer. Each juicer may have specific care instructions.

8. Replace Worn Parts:

   - Regularly check for worn or damaged parts, and promptly replace them to maintain optimal juicer performance.

9. Use Mild Cleaners:

   - When using cleaning agents, opt for mild, non-abrasive solutions to avoid damaging the juicer's components.

10. Store Properly:

    - If you're not using your juicer for an extended period, store it in its original box or cover it to protect it from dust.

Proper cleaning and maintenance are essential to ensure the longevity and efficiency of your juicer. Following these steps and tips will help you keep your juicer in top condition, allowing you to enjoy fresh and nutritious juices for a long time.

Longevity of your juicer

Extending the Longevity of Your Juicer:

1. Regular Cleaning:

- Importance: Cleaning your juicer immediately after each use prevents residue buildup, which can lead to deterioration.

- Tip: Establish a routine of thorough cleaning to keep components in optimal condition.

2. Proper Disassembly:

- Importance: Incorrect disassembly can lead to wear and tear. Following the manufacturer's instructions ensures components are handled appropriately.
- Tip: Refer to the user manual for proper disassembly steps.

**3. Gentle Handling of Parts:
- Importance: Vigorous handling can damage delicate components like the mesh screen or cutting blades.

- **Tip**: Use gentle pressure when cleaning and avoid abrasive tools.

4. Avoid Overloading:
- Importance: Overloading the juicer may strain the motor, leading to premature wear.
- Tip: Follow recommended capacity guidelines to ensure smooth operation.

5. Lubrication of Moving Parts:
- Importance: Regular lubrication of moving parts maintains efficiency and reduces friction.

- Tip: Follow manufacturer
  recommendations for lubricating
  gears or moving components.

6. Proper Storage:

- Importance: Storing the juicer in a
  cool, dry place protects it from
  environmental factors.
- Tip: Cover the juicer when not in
  use to prevent dust accumulation.

7. Avoiding Hard Ingredients:

- Importance: Hard ingredients can
  put strain on the motor and
  blades.

- Tip: Pre-cut hard items like large carrots or beets into smaller, manageable pieces.

8. Use Fresh Produce:

- Importance: Juicing fresh and ripe produce ensures a smoother process, reducing stress on the juicer.
- Tip: Avoid using overly firm or unripe fruits and vegetables.

9. Periodic Blade Maintenance:

- Importance: Dull blades can affect juicing efficiency and strain the motor.

- Tip: Sharpen or replace blades as recommended by the manufacturer.

10. Avoiding Excessive Force:

- Importance: Applying excessive force during juicing can strain components.
- Tip: Allow the juicer to process ingredients naturally without pushing or forcing them.

11. Quality of Ingredients:

- Importance: Hard seeds or pits can damage cutting blades and other components.

- Tip: Remove seeds or pits before juicing, especially if your juicer is not designed to handle them.

12. Prompt Repairs:

- Importance: Addressing issues promptly prevents further damage.
- Tip: If you notice any abnormalities or performance issues, consult the user manual or contact customer support for guidance.

13. Avoiding Citrus Peel:

- Importance: Citrus peel can be abrasive and affect the juicer's components.

- Tip: Peel citrus fruits before juicing, especially if your juicer is not designed for handling peels.

14. Moderation with High-Fiber Ingredients:

- Importance: High-fiber ingredients can lead to excessive pulp, affecting the efficiency of the juicer.
- Tip: Balance high-fiber items with watery or lower-fiber options.

15. Temperature Consideration:

- Importance: Avoid continuous use for extended periods to prevent overheating.

- **Tip**: Allow the juicer to cool down between batches, especially during large juicing sessions.

By incorporating these practices into your juicing routine, you can significantly extend the longevity of your juicer, ensuring that it continues to provide fresh and nutritious juices for an extended period.

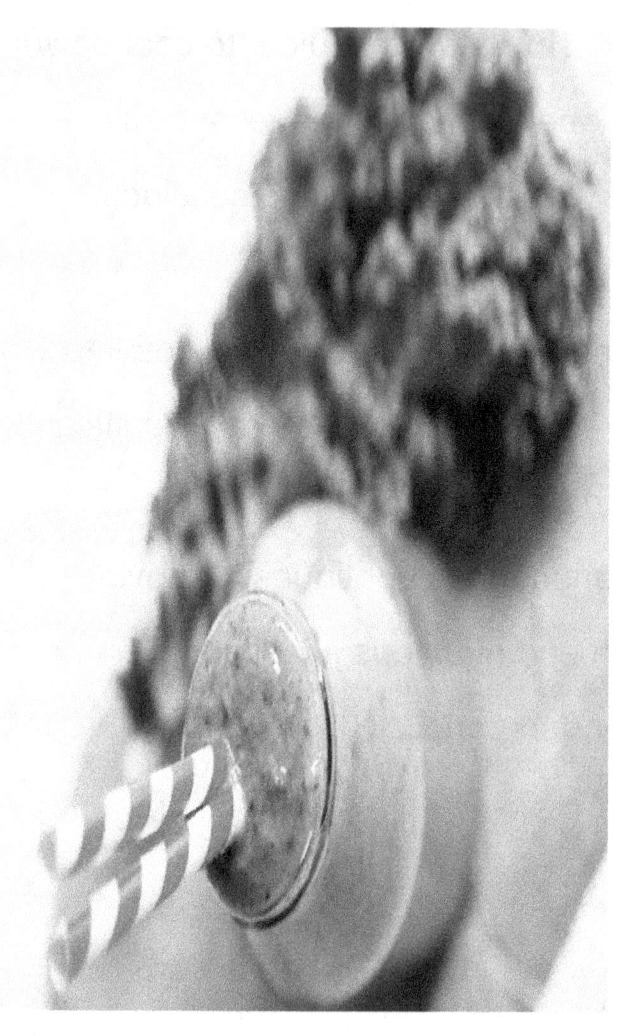

Chapter Seven

Delicious Juicing Recipes:

1. Energizing Citrus Blend:

Ingredients:

- 2 Oranges (peeled)
- 1 Grapefruit (peeled)
- 1 Lemon (peeled)
- 1 Lime (peeled)
- 2 Carrots (cleaned and trimmed)
- 1 inch Ginger (peeled)

Instructions:

1. Prepare all ingredients by peeling and trimming as necessary.

2. Feed the oranges, grapefruit, lemon, lime, carrots, and ginger into the juicer chute.

3. Juice the ingredients, ensuring a smooth blend.

4. Stir the juice to combine flavors evenly.

5. Pour the vibrant citrus blend into a glass and enjoy the refreshing burst of energy.

2. Green Goddess Detox:

Ingredients:

- 2 Green Apples (cored and sliced)

- 1 Cucumber (peeled if not organic)

- Handful of Kale

- Handful of Spinach

- 1 Celery Stalk

- 1 Lemon (peeled)

- Small bunch of Mint Leaves

Instructions:

1. Prep the green apples, cucumber, kale, spinach, celery, lemon, and mint leaves.

2. Insert each ingredient into the juicer, ensuring even distribution.

3. Juice the mixture until you achieve a vibrant green elixir.

4. Pour the detoxifying juice into a glass.

5. Garnish with a mint sprig and savor the invigorating Green Goddess Detox.

Tips for Delicious Juicing:

1. Play with Ratios:

    ○ Adjust ingredient ratios to suit your taste preferences. Trying several things will help you discover the ideal balance.

2. Chill Ingredients:

    ○ Chill fruits and vegetables before juicing for a refreshing and crisp result.

3. Add Citrus for Zing:

    - Citrus fruits like lemons and limes add a zesty kick to your juices. Adjust quantities based on your preferred level of tanginess.

4. Experiment with Herbs:

    - Herbs like mint, basil, or cilantro can elevate the flavor profile. Start with small amounts and adjust to taste.

5. Incorporate Hydrating Cucumbers:

    - Cucumbers are hydrating and contribute to a lighter texture. Include them for a refreshing twist.

6. Mindful Sweeteners:

- If you desire additional sweetness, consider natural sweeteners like honey or agave syrup. Use sparingly to maintain a healthy balance.

7. Serve Over Ice:

   - Pour your juices over ice for a chilled and satisfying experience, especially during warm weather.

8. Garnish Creatively:

   - Garnish your juices with slices of fruit, a sprig of mint, or a twist of citrus for visual appeal.

9. Prevent Oxidation:

- o Drink your juices promptly to prevent oxidation and retain maximum nutritional benefits.

10. Personalize Your Recipes:

- o Customize these recipes based on your preferences. Add or subtract ingredients to create your signature blends.

These juicing recipes are not only delicious but also packed with nutrients to support your well-being. Feel free to get creative, adapt the recipes to your taste, and enjoy the vibrant flavors of fresh, homemade juices.

Setting realistic goals and incorporating juicing into daily life

Setting realistic goals for juicing and seamlessly incorporating it into daily life involves thoughtful planning and gradual adjustments. Here's a comprehensive guide:

1. Understand Your Objectives:
   - Clarify why you want to incorporate juicing into your routine. Whether it's for

increased energy, weight
management, or overall
health, having a clear
purpose will guide your
goals.

2. Start Gradually:

   o Begin with achievable goals,
   like juicing two to three times
   a week. This allows you to
   adapt without overwhelming
   your routine.

3. Invest in a Quality Juicer:

   o Choose a juicer that aligns
   with your needs and lifestyle.
   Easy-to-clean and efficient
   machines make the process
   more enjoyable.

4. Experiment with Recipes:

   o Explore various fruit and
     vegetable combinations to
     find flavors you enjoy. This
     adds variety and prevents
     monotony.

5. Establish a Routine:

   o Incorporate juicing into your
     daily schedule, whether it's a
     morning ritual or an
     afternoon snack.
     Consistency fosters habit.

6. Prep Ingredients Ahead:

   o Wash, chop, and store fruits
     and vegetables in advance
     for quick and convenient
     juicing. This minimizes

barriers to incorporating it
daily.

7. Balanced Nutrition:

   - While juicing can offer a
     nutrient boost, it's essential
     to maintain a balanced diet.
     Ensure you're still
     consuming whole foods and
     a variety of nutrients.

8. Portion Control:

   - Pay attention to portion
     proportions to prevent
     consuming too many
     calories and sugar. A
     standard serving is typically
     around 8-16 ounces.

9. Listen to Your Body:

- Pay attention to how your body responds to juicing. Adjust your goals based on your energy levels, digestion, and overall well-being.

10. Educate Yourself:

- Learn about the nutritional content of different fruits and vegetables. This knowledge helps you create juices tailored to your specific health goals.

11. Set Realistic Frequency:

- As your body adjusts, consider increasing the frequency of juicing. Find a balance that aligns with your lifestyle and preferences.

12. Monitor Progress:

   o Track your juicing habits and how they impact your health goals. Adjust your routine as needed, keeping in mind that flexibility is key to sustainability.

13. Celebrate Milestones:

   o Acknowledge and celebrate achievements along the way. Whether it's sticking to a routine for a month or discovering a new favorite recipe, small victories reinforce positive habits.

14. Stay Hydrated:

- While juicing contributes to hydration, ensure you're still drinking an adequate amount of water throughout the day.

By combining these strategies, you can create a realistic and sustainable approach to juicing that seamlessly integrates into your daily life while supporting your health and wellness goals.

Conclusion

In conclusion, venturing into the realm of juicing as a beginner unveils a pathway to enhanced well-being and nutritional empowerment. As you navigate this exciting journey, several key considerations can shape a rewarding and sustainable experience.

Commencing with a gradual approach is fundamental. Beginners should ease into juicing, commencing with a few sessions per week and progressively scaling up. This measured initiation ensures a smooth integration into daily life without overwhelming adjustments.

Investing in a quality juicer emerges as a pivotal step. Selecting a juicing apparatus that aligns with your preferences and lifestyle streamlines the process, transforming it into an enjoyable and efficient endeavor. Whether opting for a centrifugal, masticating, or triturating juicer, the right equipment makes a substantial difference.

Diversity in juicing recipes becomes a canvas for exploration. Experimentation with a variety of fruits, vegetables, and even herbs introduces a spectrum of flavors and nutritional benefits. This creative aspect not only elevates the enjoyment of juicing but also broadens the spectrum of essential nutrients incorporated into your diet.

Consistency, established through routine, is the bedrock of a successful juicing endeavor. Integrating juicing into your daily rituals, whether as a refreshing morning routine or an afternoon energy booster, solidifies this healthy habit over time.

Understanding the importance of nutritional balance is paramount. While juicing provides a concentrated source of vitamins and minerals, it should complement, not replace, a well-rounded diet. Supplementing juices with a variety of whole foods ensures a comprehensive and balanced nutritional intake.

Portion control emerges as a guiding principle. Being mindful of the quantity consumed helps prevent excess caloric and sugar intake. Striking a balance between satiety and nutritional benefits typically involves servings ranging from 8 to 16 ounces.

In essence, the journey into juicing for beginners is an exciting exploration of flavors, nutrients, and well-being. By incorporating these principles – gradual progression, quality equipment, diverse recipes, consistency, nutritional balance, and mindful portions – beginners can carve out a fulfilling and sustainable juicing routine that aligns seamlessly with their health goals. Cheers to a vibrant and healthful juicing journey

9 7988 79 1 3 0 8 3 6